The Little Tea Handbook

Written by: Christie Elene Mogensen

Content

I say let the world go to hell, but I should always have my tea 😉
Fyodor Dostoevsky
(1821 – 1881)

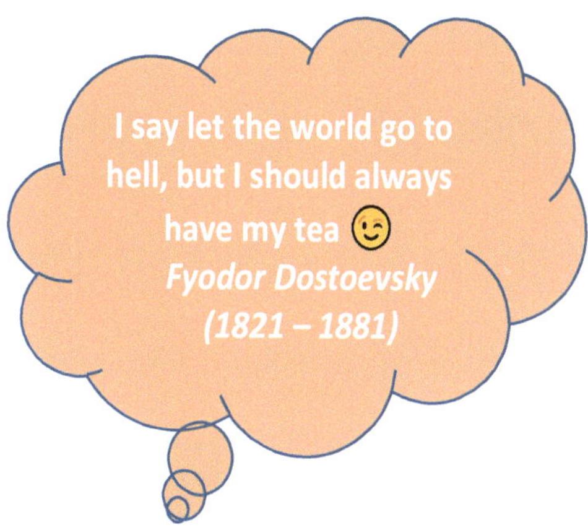

In this little handbook you will find some basic information about tea.

You will get to know about the differences between the types of tea, which tea might be the best for you and you will find out why tea is so amazing.

Also you'll find out how to brew a good cup of tea and how to use the tea leaves as a snack or maybe a drink. All of this is presented in an easy-going way.

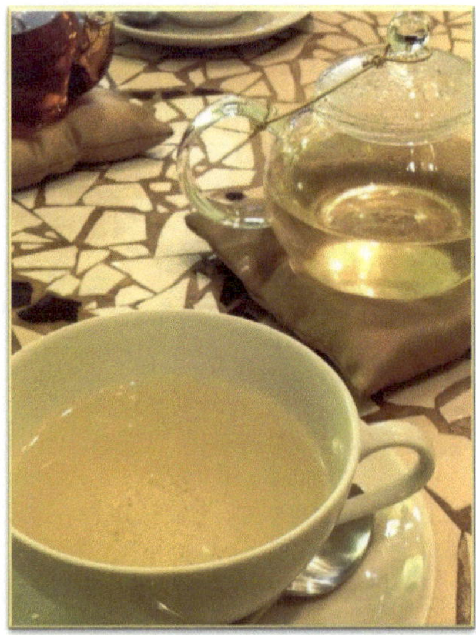

There is also get a short introduction to our web-site 'Organic Tea'.

About me

I am a young Dane living in Copenhagen, who is very environmentally conscious and drinks tea most of the day.

It all started with a blog in Copenhagen. Having had a passion for tea for several years, I got the idea to create a blog with tea as the main focus.

My spouse Mogens supplemented with his idea of creating a tea database. Thus, Organic-tea.org was born!

At our web-site www.organic-tea.org you will find the worlds first and largest collection of organic teas!

If you, like us, believe that organic farming is the future, take a look at our web-site www.organic-tea.org.

Why not go organic with us? 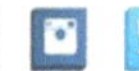

1.1 Short introduction to Organic Tea

We have carefully selected teas and created the world's first and largest collection of different brands of organic teas.

At Organic Tea you can select between:

- ✓ 20+ wonderful brands
- ✓ 70+ flavour selections
- ✓ 10+ wellbeing options, including bedtime tea, relaxing tea, ayurvedic tea, breastfeeding mother's tea etc.
- ✓ Gift packages
- ✓ Christmas Advent Calendars

You can also find the most adorable teaware and products related to tea such as:

- Tea pots

- Tea cups

- Tea strainers

- Tea cosys

- Tea canisters

- Tea warmers

- Matcha bowls

- Books about tea

- Steam Wavers

- Other teaware

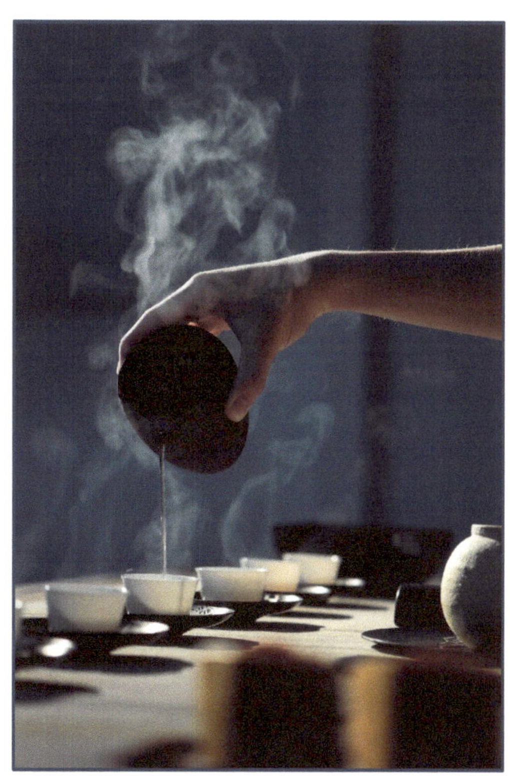

The world's oldest cultivated plant is believed to be the tea plant Camellia Sinensis, which has been grown in China for about 2500 years.

It is said, however, that the tea plant was already known 5000 years ago. The oldest reliable information is from the year 221 B.C., where scrolls documenting the introduction of a new tax on tea were found.

Tea is served in China at every meal – before the food as a refreshment, and after dinner to help digestion.

Emperor Shen Nung discovered tea

There are many stories about how tea was actually discovered.

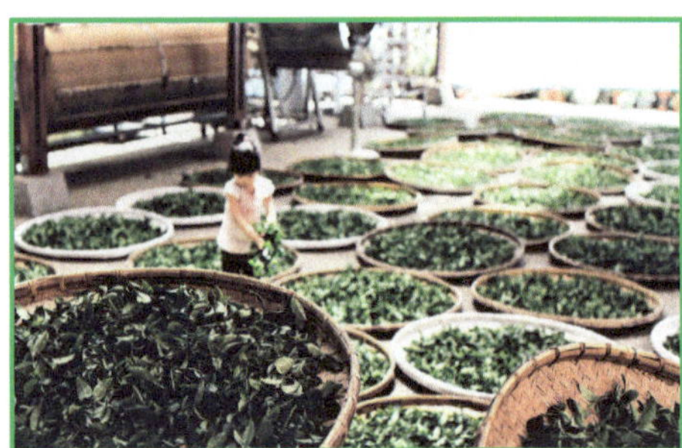

According to legend, the Emperor Shen Nung (2737-2697 b. c.), who drank boiled water for health reasons, discovered tea.

One day some leaves blew from a tea plant into his cup and coloured the water. The Emperor liked the smell, and was curious. He tasted the coloured water, and found it refreshing.

The Emperor was so excited about his new discovery that he started the first tea production, and a long tradition was thus born.

The road to Europe

In the 1500's the knowledge of tea and the properties of tea came to Europe with missionaries and sailors. Trade with tea started when Dutch merchants in 1610 brought the tea to Amsterdam.

Tea came to America in the mid-1600's

Dutchman Peter Stuyvesant brought the first tea to America to the colonists in the Dutch settlement of New Amsterdam (later re-named New York by the English).

Do you find it difficult to navigate through the many thousands of different kinds of tea?

A good way to help you into this universe is to divide tea into two main types:

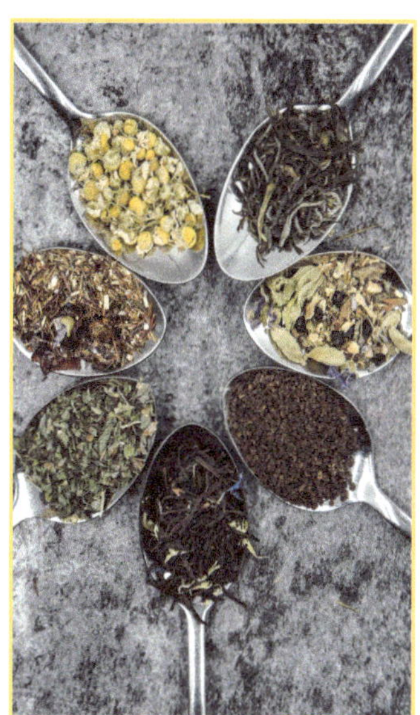

- tea from the tea plant 'Camellia Sinensis' – such as black tea, green tea, white tea etc.
- tea from all plants other - e.g. tisanes/herbal teas

Today these teas are produced from the tea plant Camellia Sinensis:

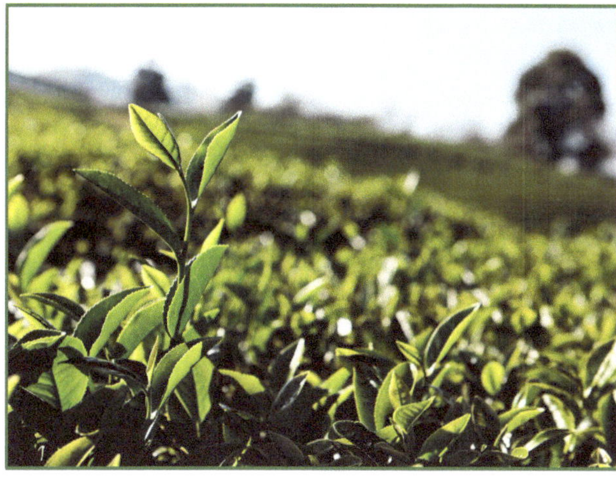

Black tea
Green tea
White tea
Oolong tea
Pu-erh tea
Yellow tea
Matcha

Tea which does not come from the tea plant Camellia Sinensis, may be for example chamomile tea, rooibos tea or Greek mountain tea. These teas have other health benefits than tea from Camellia Sinensis.

In the following chapters I will only focus on tea from the tea plant Camellia Sinensis and briefly describe the differences between black tea, green tea, white tea, oolong tea, pu-erh tea, yellow tea and matcha.

4.1 Introduction

The tea plant called Camellia Sinensis produces the leaves and buds that are commonly known as tea – the most common beverage consumed in the world, second only to water.

How the leaves from Camellia Sinensis are processed will determine their final classification as black tea, green tea, white tea or oolong tea etc.

According to Chinese Medicine, tea possesses various properties depending on the type of tea.

Discover which tea suits you the best!

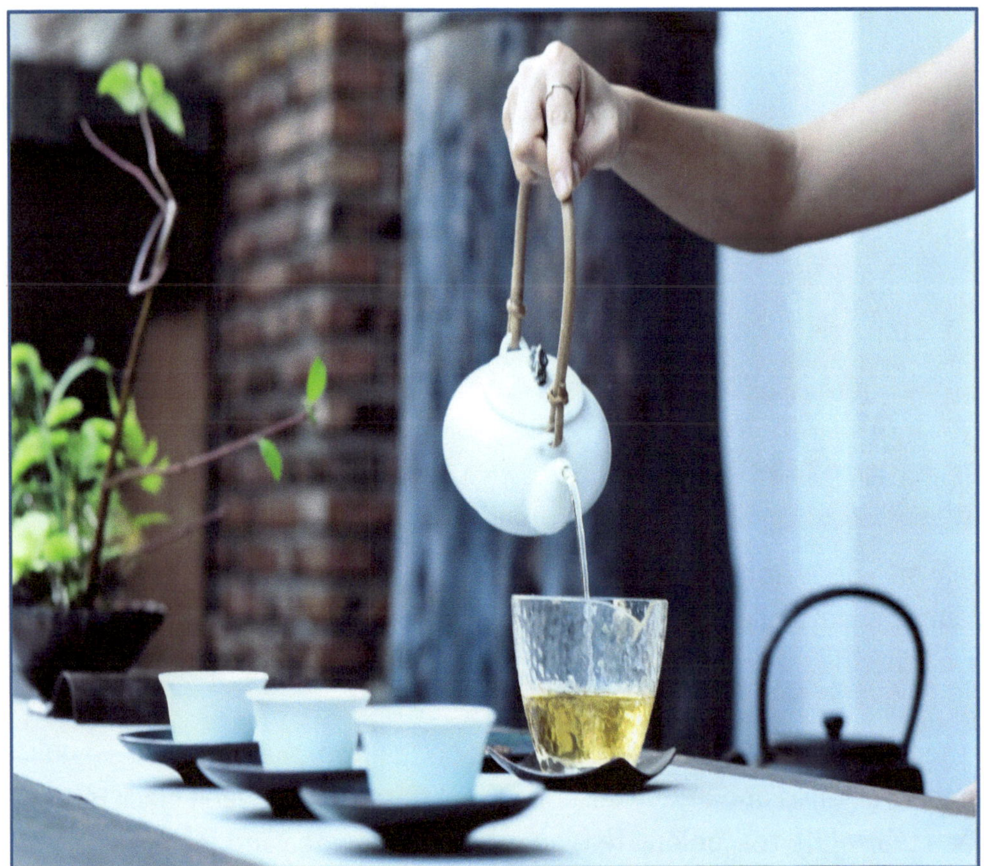

4.2 Black Tea

Black tea is the most common type of tea in the West. The main reason is because black tea was the tea type, that was imported to Europe and later the U.S. in the 1600's.

Black tea is fully oxidized*, has a stronger flavor and a higher caffeine content in general than other teas from the tea plant.

Drinking black tea offers a variety of health benefits, as it contains antioxidants and compounds that have the ability to affect the body in a very beneficial way.

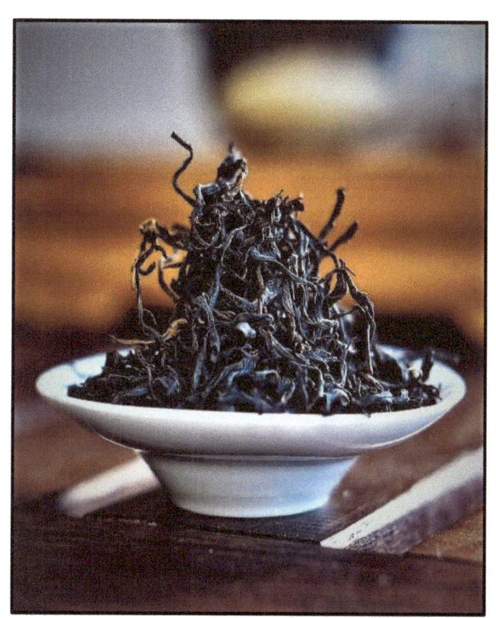

Among other it sets digestion into action, expands blood vessels, and strengthens the heart.

According to traditional Chinese medicine, black tea is most suitable for those living in cold climates because it warms and nourishes the body.

The process of making black tea:

1. First allowing the tea leaves to wither

2. Then they are rolled or crushed by hand or machine

3. This activates the oxidation processes and the tea leaves turn black

4. Finally, they are fired in ovens to stop the oxidation process

* Oxidation is a chemical reaction that alters the flavour of the tea leaves and helps the processed tea develop its ultimate appearance and colour.

4.3 Green Tea

Green tea has been consumed in China for at least 2000 years, and it was surprisingly not the first tea to be produced. It is (still) the most popular tea in Asia, almost as popular as coffee is in the West.

In China drinking green tea daily is recommended for the support of a healthy lifestyle.

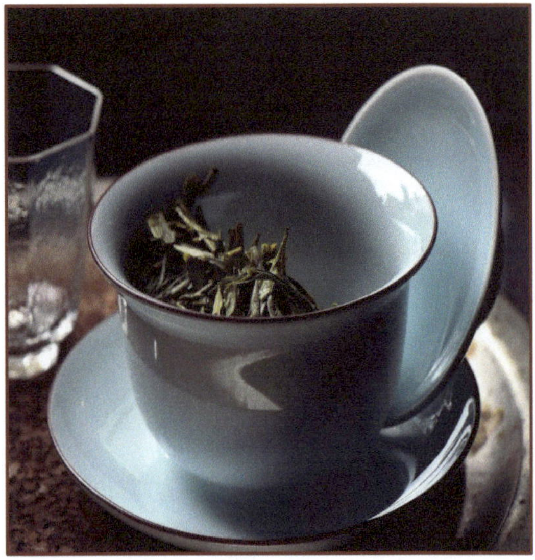

According to traditional Chinese medicine green tea has a cooling effect, even though it is a warm drink. Green tea is also thought to relax your liver, reduce the risk of cancer, improve your mood, reduce stress and increase energy.

In general, green tea is associated with a lot of beneficial health effects. This is mainly due to the variant of the catechins called EGCG (more about EGCG at page 20).

There are countless varieties of green tea, all with their own shape, appearance and taste profile. Green tea is generally grassy with a taste of vegetables.

The process of making green tea:

1. First allowing the tea leaves to wither

2. Tea leaves are now ready to be either fried (the Chinese method) or steamed (the Japanese method)

3. After heat treatment, the tea is shaped while it is still warm and supple

4. The shaped green tea leaves are then left to dry

4.4 White Tea

White tea is the closest you can get to the naturally untreated tea leaves.

White tea has a limited harvest season, as it can only be picked in the early spring, when the young buds are still covered by fine white hairs, hence the name 'white' tea.

As white tea is not heat-treated, all the vitamins are retained in the buds. Fresh white tea has about three times as many antioxidants as most green teas.

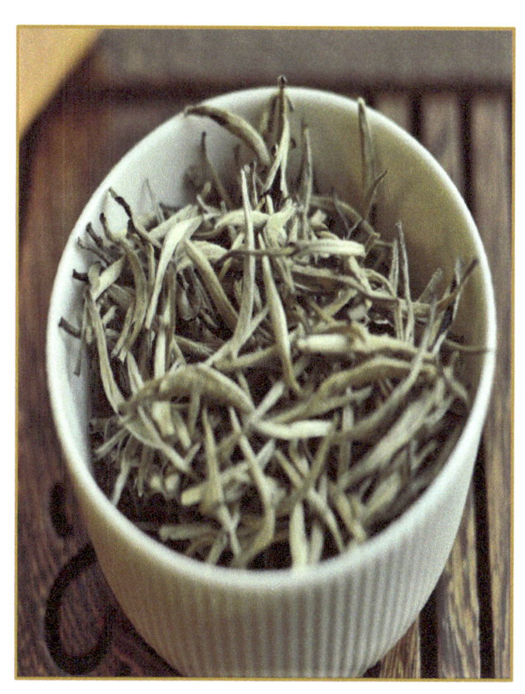

In China, white tea is used to reduce body temperature, to counteract fluid accumulation and stimulate the intestinal tract.

White tea has a mild and slightly sweet flavour and lacks the grassy flavour you often find in green tea.

The process of making white tea:

1. As soon as the buds are plucked, they are allowed to wither and air dry in the sun or in a carefully controlled outdoor or indoor environment.

2. This minimal processing and low oxidation result in some of the most delicate and freshest tea available.

4.5 Oolong Tea

Oolong tea is semi-oxidized, which places it between black and green tea. Each type of oolong tea has a different manufacturing process related to the area in which it is grown.

For tea-enthusiasts oolong tea is probably the most sought after of all types of tea, as it is a tea that offers a wide range of aromas with sophisticated and refined flavors.

In China, the more oxidized oolong teas are used to help cure headaches, and cleanse the body after excessive intake of toxins such as cigarettes and alcohol.

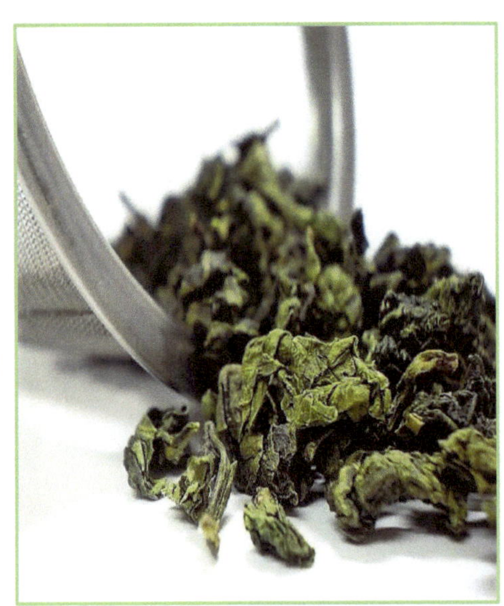

In recent years, oolong tea has also attracted attention as it is recognized as a weight loss tea that decreases body fat and speeds up metabolism.

The process of making oolong tea in general:

1. First allowing the tea leaves to wither

2. After withering a light rolling process helps the tea leaves develop their unique appearance and flavour profile

3. Then the tea leaves are allowed to oxidize. Oolong teas vary in levels of oxidation, anywhere from 8% to 80%

4. To halt the oxidation process and to start drying out the leaves, heat is applied

5. A key characteristic of any oolong is its shape, so before the final rolling begins, the leaves are shaped

6. The shaped oolong tea leaves are then left to dry

4.6 Pu-erh tea

Pu-erh tea is a fermented, aged tea that comes from the Yunnan province of China. It is one of China's most famous medical teas, and it has been enjoyed for more than a thousand years.

Just like wine, Pu-erh tea is thought to get better with age!

In traditional Chinese medicine Pu-erh tea has long been valued for its ability to:

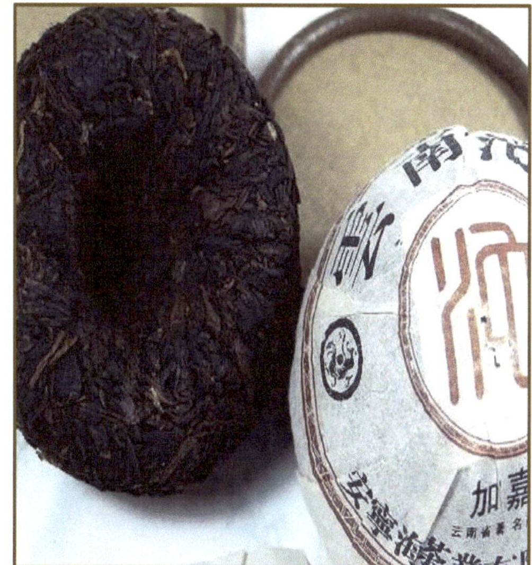

- lower blood sugar
- boost immunity,
- lower cholesterol
- increase energy
- promote a healthy heart
- reduce stress
- prevent illness etc. etc.

Pu-erh tea is regularly categorized as a slim tea.
Scientific studies periodically reveal new results such as Pu-erh tea increases fat burning and decreases the body's ability to absorb fat.

Pu-erh tea has a deep, distinctive and earthy taste.

It comes in two varieties: green (sheng) and black (shou), depending on how the leaves are fermented.

The process of making Pu-Erh tea in general:

1. Sun-withered leaves are put into a wok and fired
2. After cooling, they are handrolled in order to break down the cells to release flavour

3. Pu-erh leaves are then sun-dried
4. This results in a raw tea, called maocha, which can be made for either sheng or shou Pu-erh tea
5. Sheng Pu-erh is steamed and pressed into cakes and allowed to ferment naturally via microbial bacteria
6. Shu Pu-erh undergoes fermentation called wet piling. The tea is piled in mounds and water is added. As the tea begins to ferment the tea is turned until it is completely black
7. Both varieties are then stored for aging for at least one year

As Sheng Pu-erh tea is naturally stored and evolves over time, it is considered to be the finest Pu-erh tea, highly sought after by tea lovers all over the world.

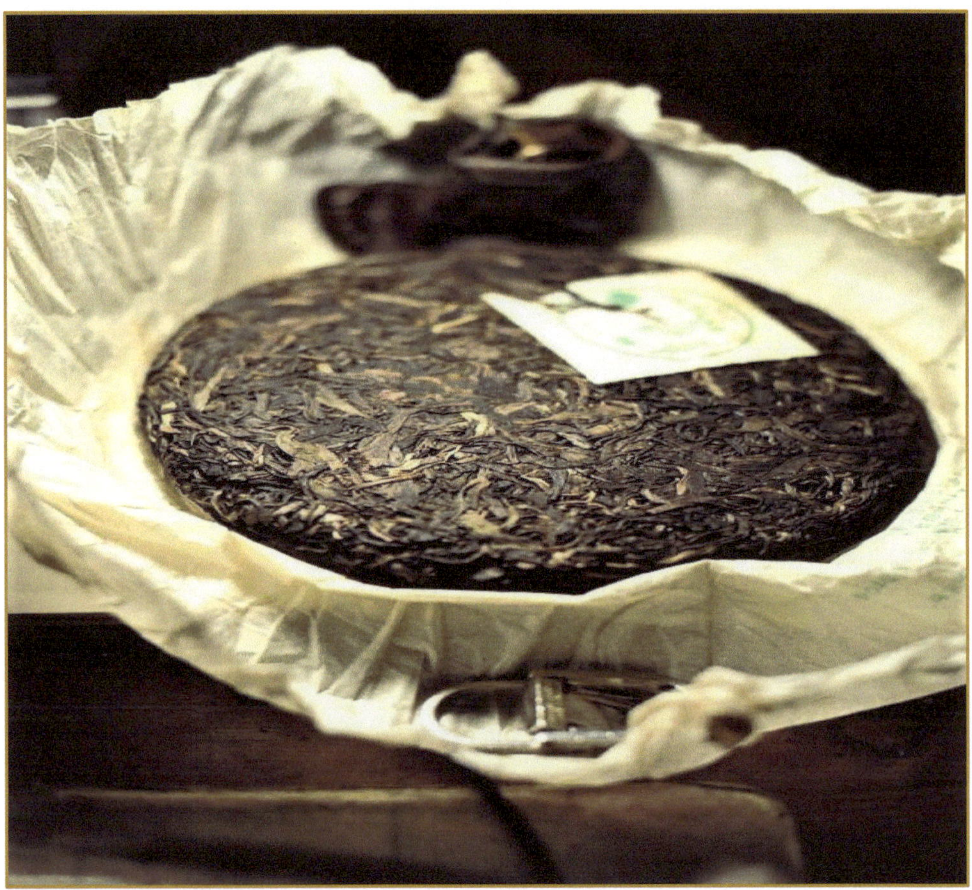

4.7 Yellow tea

Yellow tea is a very rare type of tea and therefore one of the most expensive teas in the world. It is a speciality of Anhui, Sichuan, Zhejiang and Hunan provinces in China.

There are just a handful of famous yellow teas in China and the production is very limited. Yellow tea was often, historically, used as a tribute tea, given as a gift to the emperor.

For people with sensitive stomachs, yellow tea is often a more milder tea than green tea.

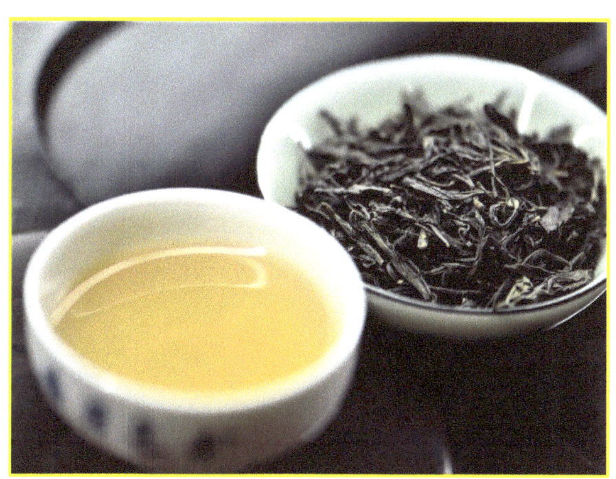

Due to its slow fermentation process, yellow tea is considered by many to be very beneficial to the spleen and stomach.

The process for making yellow tea is time consuming.

Here is the process in general:

1. The leaves are first fried, as is the case in most green teas

2. Then the leaves are wrapped in thick paper or linen cloth

3. The leaves are allowed to damp, which gives the tea a slight fermentation. At intervals the tea is cooled and re-wrapped until the leaves becomes dry

4. This process can continue for up to three days

4.8 Matcha tea

Matcha is a Japanese word meaning powdered tea.

Ever since the 13th century, Matcha tea has been part of the Japanese tea tradition and even to this day Matcha is one of the most prized beverages in Japan.

Drinking one cup of Matcha tea is equivalent to about 7 cups of green tea. As you're basically ingesting the whole leaf rather than the infusion.

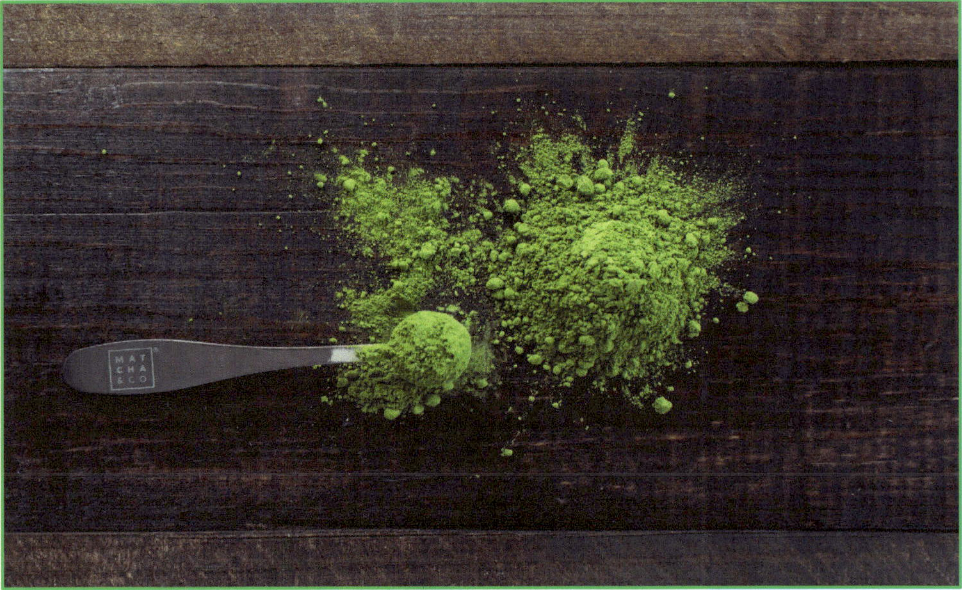

Matcha tea is a very powerful superfood as it is packed with antioxidants, fibre, vitamins, minerals and mood-lifting elements.

Due to the high chlorophyll content Matcha is also believed to act as a powerful detoxifier that can remove heavy metals from your body.

Besides health benefits such as decreasing the risk of heart disease, cancer and liver disease, don't forget that Matcha tea also seems to have an impact on your metabolism and on your weight.

The process of making Matcha powder:

1. The tea leaves undergo a shading process two to six weeks before harvest time, where they are covered by bamboo mats or rice straws mounted on top. By covering the leaves from direct sunlight, the amounts of both chlorophyll and L-theanine (look at page 18) are increasing

2. Only first flush leaves from the top of the plant – two leaves and an open bud are picked

3. The freshly picked leaves are steamed and dried, ribs and stems removed, leaving only the soft leaf tissue, called tencha

4. Tencha is then kept refrigerated until it is ready to be ground

5. Tea processors grind the tencha on a stonemill in order to achieve a fine, smooth powder texture and superior consistency

Matcha workshop in Copenhagen

If you are visiting Copenhagen, try a Matcha workshop at Sing Tehus, Kompagnistræde 30.

It's so nice to meet others who share the passion for tea.

The Matcha workshop is both fun and informative. You get a little talk first, and afterwards you are allowed to whip your own Matcha.

Matcha workshop takes place from 11 am to 12.30 pm, the first Saturday of each month.

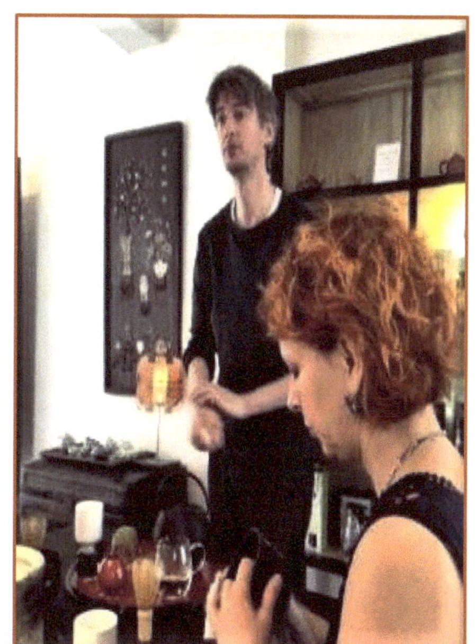

The fact that tea (from the tea plant Camellia Sinensis) makes you feel better sounds like a cliché. But this cliché "has a name". It is called L-theanine.

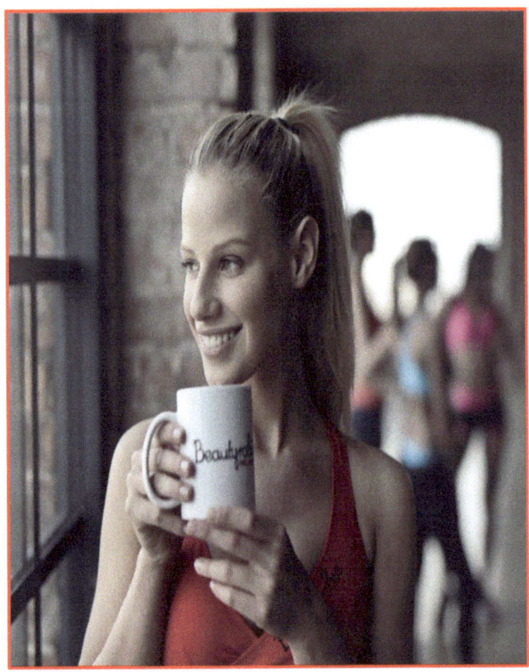

L-theanine is an amino acid* that so far is only found in tea leaves, an inedible mushroom and an Amazonian tree. Therefore, tea is the most natural way to get a good dose of L-theanine.

L-theanine boosts your mood and reduces stress. It has also been proven to have many positive effects on humans such as triggering the release of alpha-waves which enhances creativity, focus and relaxation.

Even low levels of L-theanine have demonstrated altered brain wave states (alpha waves) inducing relaxation.

Other than that, it has been shown to improve cognition, learning, remembering skills, concentration, promote faster simple reaction time and faster numeric working memory reaction time.

In addition, L-theanine has been shown to help boost our white blood cell count, which is another way to prevent illness.

* Amino acids are the building blocks of proteins. Proteins are necessary for many of the structures and functions in our bodies.

5.1 Teas high in L-theanine

If you are buying your tea at the supermarket, don't expect it to be filled with L-theanine.

There are several factors that determine the levels of L-theanine, such as how and where the tea is grown and when the tea is harvested.

Tea harvested early in the spring <u>and</u> protected from sunlight (sunlight transforms the L-theanine into polyphenols) contains most L-theanine.

These teas have the highest quality:

- ➤ Darjeeling tea, and all First Flush teas

- ➤ Silver Needle, a white tea consisting of spring buds

- ➤ Shade-grown green tea such as Gyokuro (gyokuro and Matcha are usually from the same harvest and often the same plant material)

- ➤ Matcha tea

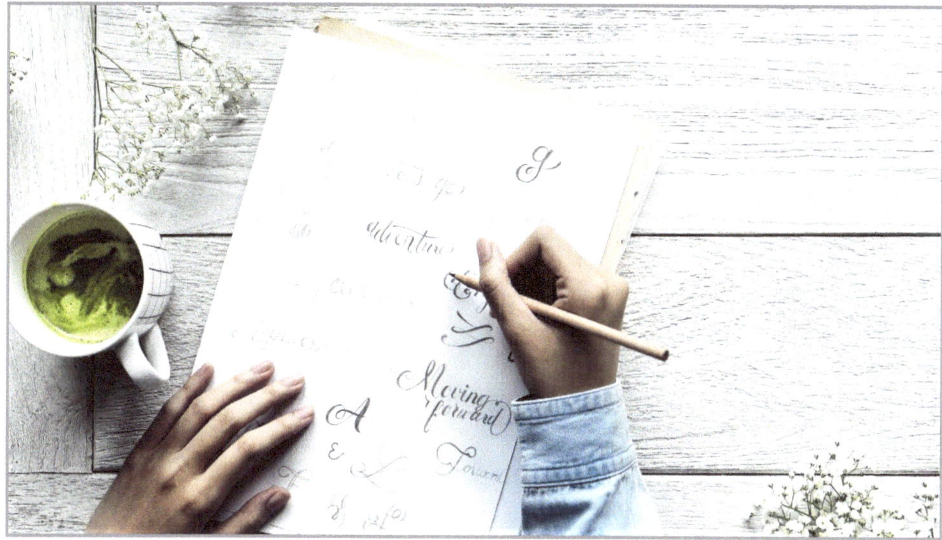

5.2 Tea (from the tea plant Camellia Sinensis) is also full of antioxidants

Tea chemistry is complex and research still has to be done to discover all of the magic in tea.

I will briefly describe some of the plant components in tea, and if you are not already convinced why you should drink more tea, maybe these facts will encourage you to.

Polyphenols

Tea contains high concentrations of polyphenols (antioxidants), which are a class of phytochemicals associated with heart disease and cancer prevention.
Polyphenols help reduce cholesterol levels, blood pressure and inhibit blood clotting.

Flavonoids

Flavonoids are a specific class of polyphenols present not only in tea, but also in fruits, vegetables and red wine.
Besides possessing strong antioxidant properties, flavonoids contribute significantly to taste and color and are considered to help maintain certain normal, healthy body functions.
Among the many benefits attributed to flavonoids are the reduced risk of cancer, heart disease, asthma, and stroke.

Catechins (EGCG)

Catechins are the primary flavonoids produced by the Camellia Sinensis plant. As green and white tea leaves undergo minimal processing, they retain the leaf's naturally high level of catechins.

EGCG (Epigallocatechin Gallate) is the main catechin in green tea and appears to be the most powerful—with antioxidant activity about 25-100 times more potent than vitamins C and E.

Catechins are believed to fight aging and cancer and are responsible for the slightly astringent, bitter flavor often associated with green tea.

In Japanese studies EGCG has shown to be highly inhibitory for the formation of lung cancer.

EGCG is one of the main reasons that smokers should drink at least three cups of green tea per day.

EGCG is also an effective means of fighting viruses, including influenza viruses which may cause high fever infections.

Chlorophyll

Chlorophyll is naturally antiseptic and has the ability to kill unwanted bacteria.

It is known to help with cleansing the body, combating infection, supporting wound healing, increasing the number of red blood cells and thereby the ability to absorb oxygen in the body.

Matcha being carefully shade-grown is substantially richer in chlorophyll than other green teas, making it a superior daily detox.

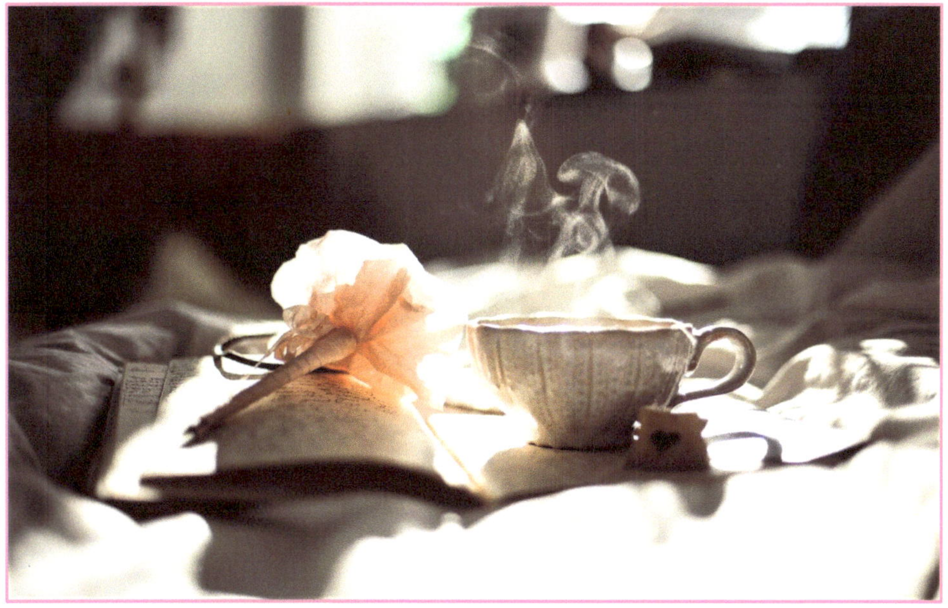

Flavored teas are created by adding fruits, flowers, herbs and other natural flavors to almost any tea type. Some of the world's most loved and popular flavored teas include:

> ➢ Earl Grey, the most popular flavored tea of Britain, prepared by adding extract of bergamot - a citrus fruit - to black tea leaves.

> ➢ Jasmine tea is tea infused with the aroma of jasmine blossoms. It is the most popular scented tea of China usually made with green tea.

The flavors complement the tea, rather than covering up the delicate aromas of the tea leaves. The main reason for flavoring tea is to obtain different blends, styles and flavors, and to create distinctive, enhanced tastes.

With roughly 70 flavours in our organic tea collection you are almost certain to find your favorite flavor.

You can also find flavor combinations you have never dreamed of:

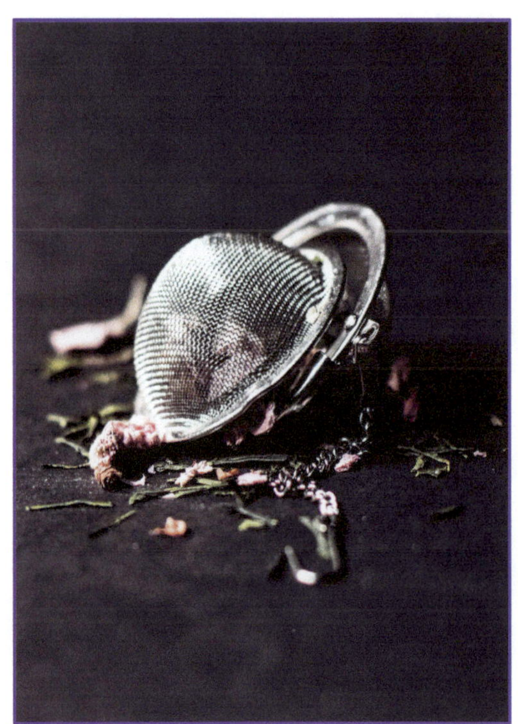

> ➢ White tea with chilli and strawberry

> ➢ Green tea with gingko and caramel flavor

> ➢ Or how about a Rooibos tea with cinnamon, ginger and coconut flakes

Always use fresh cold water from the cold tap for your tea.

Let the water run for a while first.

This ensures that you do not use water that has been laying in the pipes too long and has lost its oxygen.

Or you can use spring water. This is nice, but expensive.

Remember to throw away the bottle for recycling 😉

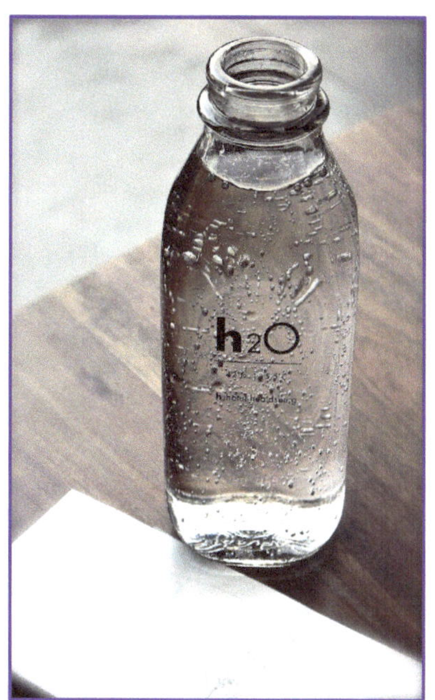

7.1 Water temperature

The water temperature means everything when you brew tea.

Various types of tea require different water temperatures.
If you want to make sure that the water has the right temperature, you can buy a kettle with a thermostat for making tea. Here you can set the exact water temperature.

Otherwise, buy a little thermometer that can measure the water temperature.

Always check the recommended water temperature for each tea.

Here are some general guidelines:

> *Black tea:* Use boiling water for black tea and short infusion time. Remove the tea leaves so your tea will not taste bitter. You can brew the same tea leaves several times, if you use good quality tea

> *Green tea:* Use water that is 80°C or 175°F. You can brew the same tea leaves several times, if you use good quality tea

> *White tea:* Use water that is 85°C – 90°C or 185°F – 194°F. You can brew the same tea leaves several times, if you use good quality tea

7.2 Room to roam

Tea leaves like to have good space.

If they are squeezed too much into a small strainer or a filter, the water will not free the aroma complex from the leaves and will therefore not extract enough flavour.

For that reason, it is important that your tea strainers or filters are big enough for the tea leaves to take up less than half the space (the leaves need to move freely).

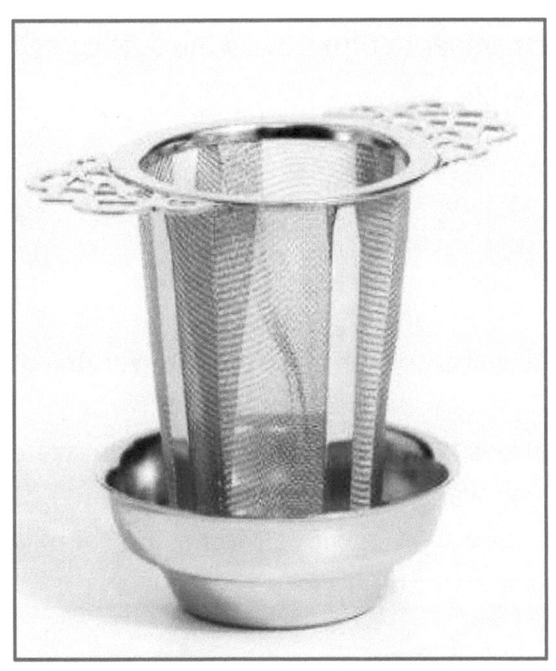

7.3 Pot and pitcher

Choose your teapot from your heart, but think about how many cups it can hold, how long it can keep warm, and what teas you want to brew.

If you invest in a nice glass pitcher, use it only for white or green tea, as it can be difficult to keep the glass pitcher clean when using it for black tea.

A glass pitcher and clear glass mugs are very suitable for tea blossoms.

7.4 The right amount of leaves

Getting the measurements correct is important for taste. For most ordinary teas you need about 2 grams of tea per 200 ml cup.

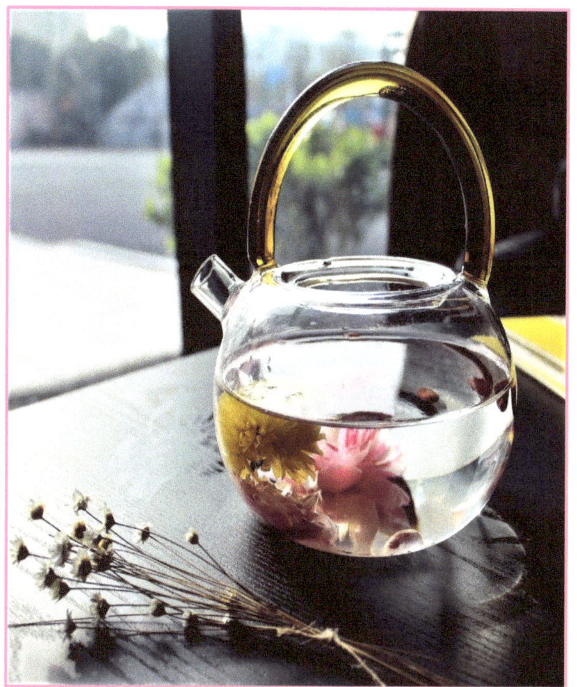

Many tend to use too few tea leaves as some teas tend to be reasonably broad-leaved and take up a lot of space compared to their weight.

If you don't use the right amount of tea and then compensate for the taste by steeping longer, you will risk brewing a bitter cup of tea.

7.5 Steeping times

The steeping time depends on the processing and size of the tea leaves.

Obviously, you must always check the recommended steeping times for each tea.

Some teas will get bitter if you don't follow the recommended steeping time. Especially the cheaper ones ☺

Your tea leaves can be used in countless ways. On the internet you can find lots of recipes using tea as a herb.

I will show you some easy recipes on how to prepare snacks, drinks and cold brewed tea.

8.1 Snacks

When your tea is brewed, you usually throw the tea leaves out. But instead of throwing them out, do as the Japanese. They make a snack based on the used tea leaves!

How to make a snack based on tea:

- Use a high-quality green tea
- Brew & drink your tea just as usual
- Put the used tea leaves in a bowl
- Pour a little bit of good soy over
- Serve!

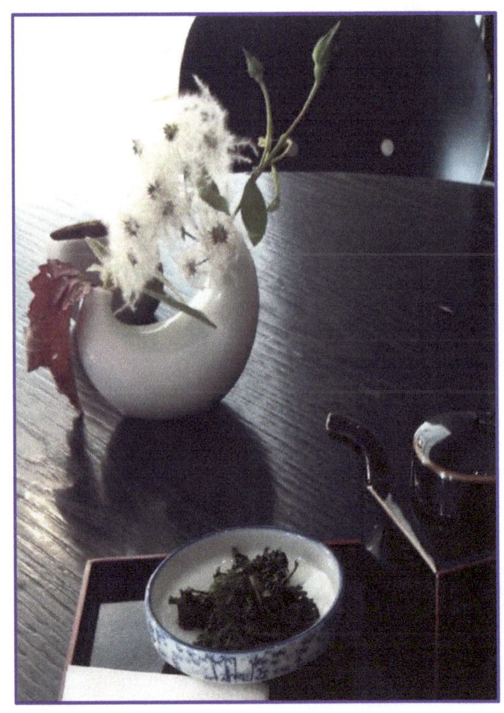

Or you can use the tea leaves along with your cooked rice.

Mix or sprinkle the tea leaves over your rice. The combination of rice and tea leaves is awesome!

Try it tonight! It is such a fun and tasty experience…

8.2 Drinks based on tea

Mixing tea in cocktails isn't new, in fact it was used to lengthen drinks in the 1800's, but it is becoming popular in bars again.

Tea works really well with gin, because it has plenty of botanical flavors to play against, whether floral or citrus.

I have tasted a few cocktails based on tea, and if you love Earl Grey like me, you have to try this very simple recipe.

Greytini

Begin by brewing a pot of Earl Grey and let it cool. Once the tea is ready, just add the rest…

Ingredients:

2 parts gin
2 parts earl grey (cold)
Squeeze of lemon
Spoonful of sugar or syrup

To make Greytini:

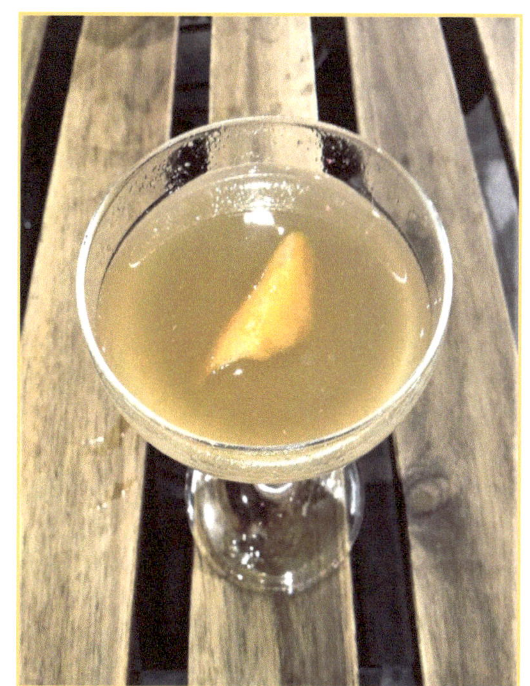

- ➢ Pour the ingredients into a martini glass filled with ice
- ➢ Stir well
- ➢ Garnish with mint leaves or lime

Cheers 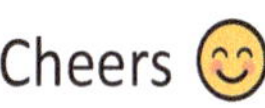

Green Apple Vodka
4 servings

This drink is mild and mouth-watering. The green tea adds a bit of
bitterness, so the drink is not too sweet.

Ingredients:

1 Granny Smith apple
2 – 3 tsp of green tea or 2
tea bags
2 cups of boiling water
1 lime, fresh squeezed
½ cup of vodka
1 cup of ginger ale
Ice cubes
Apple and lime in slices

How to make Green
Apple Vodka:

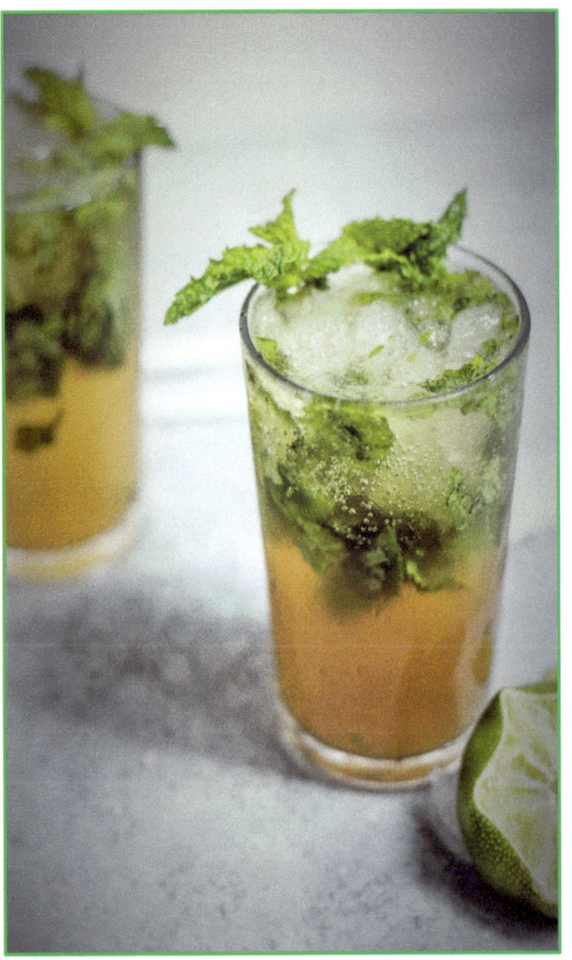

> Peel the apple and cut
  into thin boats. Pour
  the boiling water over
  the apple and tea
> Steep the tea and
  apples for about 3 – 4
  minutes, and let it
  cool completely
> Strain the tea and mix
  lime, vodka and
  ginger ale
> Serve the drink with ice cubes and slices of apple and lime

Tip! If you want your Green Apple Vodka a little sweeter, you can
sweeten with agave syrup.

8.3 Cold brewed tea

Cold brewed tea is tea steeped in cold water either in the refrigerator or at room temperature for an extended period of time. The process brews the tea leaves slowly, using time rather than temperature to release the flavors.

Cold brewed tea is known to gently extract flavors from the tea, allowing for a truer tasting tea.

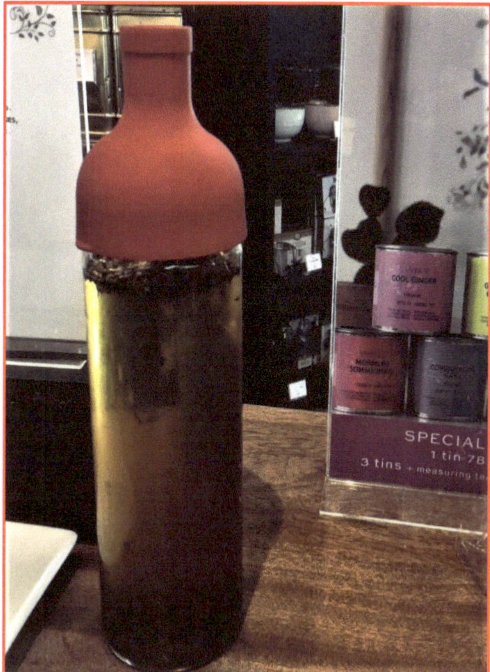

The idea of Hario Cold Brew Tea is an invitation to enjoy cold tea, just like you enjoy a glass of wine during meals.

The taste is completely different than hot tea.

Try to cold brew e.g. Kukicha tea, Japanese Bancha tea or Sencha Satsuma. Or just your favourite tea!

Herbal tea, Rooibos and Honeybush tea will also be good cold brewed.

How to brew:

- ➤ Put the leaves inside the glass tea bottle and pour on cold water

- ➤ Put the removable filter, which acts as a spout with a lid, onto the glass tea bottle

- ➤ Place it in the refrigerator and enjoy cold brew tea 3 to 6 hours later

- ➤ Pour directly from the glass tea bottle into a glass

Keep it in an airtight, dark, dry place away from strong-smelling foods.

If you buy a large amount of tea, you can divide it into what you will be using and leave the rest of it in the package.

Wrap it up in a plastic bag without air and seal it with a tight knot. Then place the airtight packaged tea somewhere dark and cool.

Tea is one of the foods that you can keep for a long time without worrying about whether it will last.

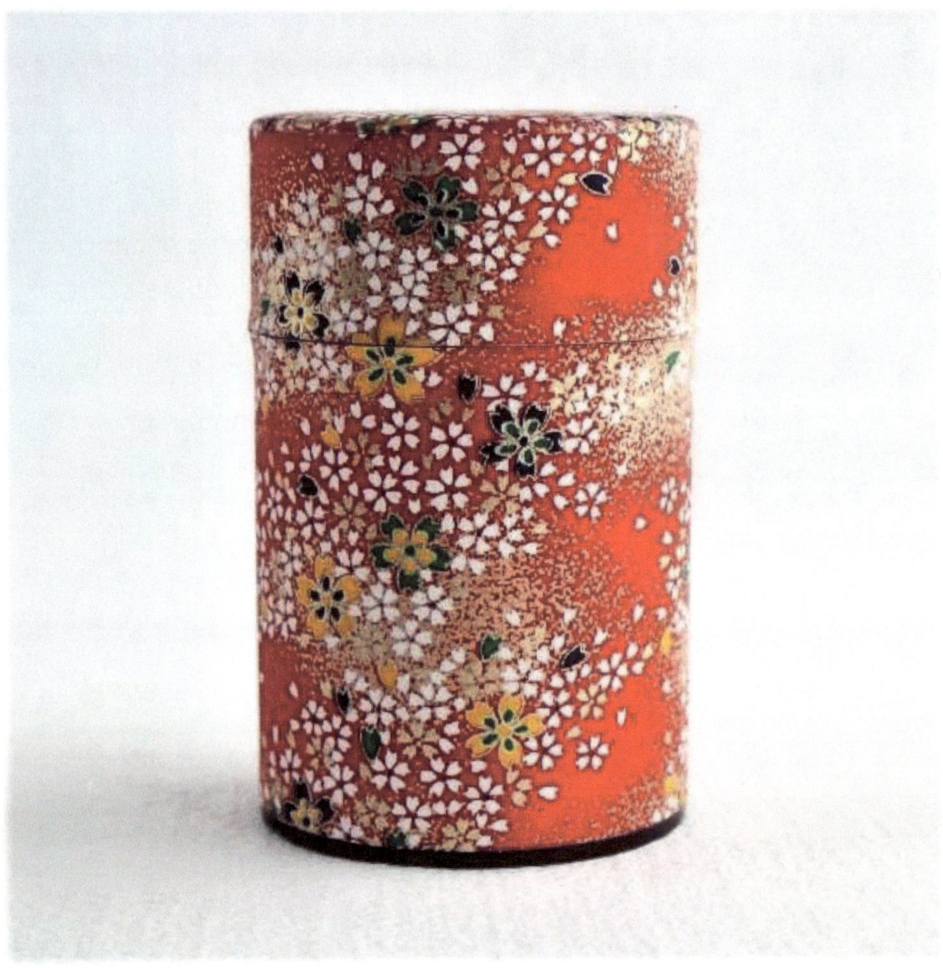

I drink a lot of tea, but never after 6 pm as tea from the teaplant Camellia Sinensis contains caffeine.

One cup of black tea contains approx. 40 mg of caffeine per cup and green tea approx. 10 mg of caffeine per cup. So, if you are as caffeine sensitive as I am, it doesn't take much for your body to react 😉

Teas from the tea plant Camellia Sinensis that I am drinking at the moment are:

Breakfast tea

My favourite breakfast tea is the Chinese black tea, called Keemun or Qimen.

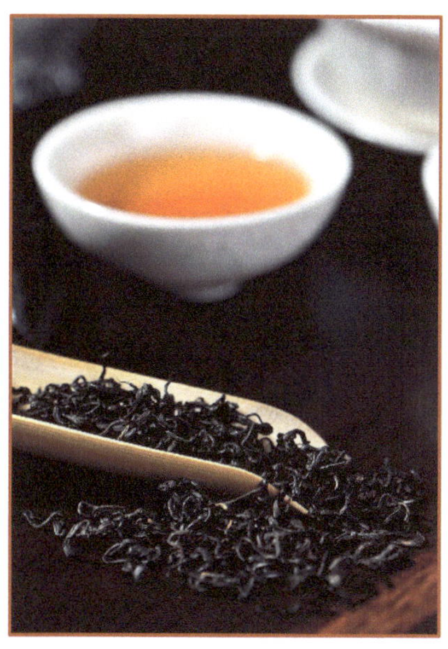

It is produced in Qimen county in the Anhui Province of China, hence the name Qimen tea.

I find Keemun tea quite tasty. It does not get bitter and it has notes of tobacco and malt with a sweet aftertaste.

Afternoon tea

In the afternoon I usually have an oolong tea. Oolong is one of my favourites as it is not as grassy as green tea.

It is a tea with a wide range of different oxidation levels, aromas and flavors ranging from fruity to floral. Oolong tea can have complex notes of nuts, butter, chocolate and roasted sugar.

The herbal teas I prefer in the evening are all without caffeine

<u>Greek Mountain tea</u>

I like drinking Greek Mountain tea with a dash of lemon & honey.

Greek Mountain tea has a mild, smooth and slightly sweet taste and can be enjoyed cold as well as hot.

It is said to boost the immune system and has been found to have antibacterial, antiviral, anti-inflammatory and antioxidative properties.

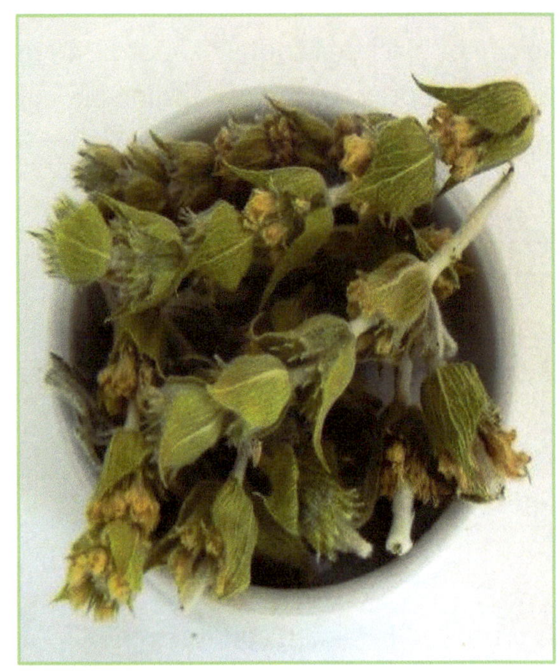

In addition, it tastes just fantastic!

<u>Herbal infusion with valerian</u>

At the moment I am also drinking an herbal infusion called 'Meditate' by the British brand 'Hampstead Tea'.

Meditate is an organic blend of lemongrass, oat flowers, lavender and valerian root.

Valerian is excellent when you want to calm down and it is often referred to as 'nature's Valium' known for its magical ability to relax your body and help you sleep better.

In other words, a really good bedtime tea!

Rooibos tea

I first got to know about rooibos tea, when a beautiful African man served the tea to me in South Africa 15 years ago.

Rooibos is one of my favourite bedtime teas, with its smooth, sweet and nutty taste.

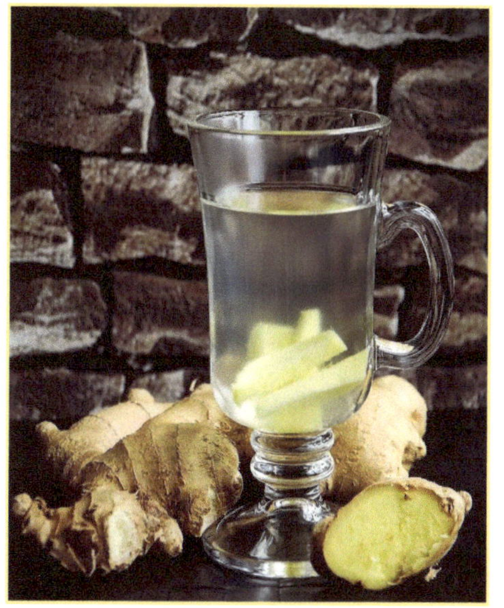

It is packed with antioxidants including two antioxidants both contributing to stress reducing effects, which is why rooibos tea is a very soothing and useful evening tea.

Ginger tea

Make your very own home-brewed ginger tea. For one cup of tea:

- Boil water and allow to cool slightly for approx. 185°F
- Finely cut some slices of ginger and pour the hot water over them
- Let it sit for at least 4 - 5 minutes and season with a little honey

Deliciously refreshing and also suitable for iced tea.

Besides being a tea nerd, I love meaningful quotes.

My favorite philosopher is Rumi - one of the greatest poets who wrote about life, love and spirituality.

Who is Rumi

He is an Influential Persian poet who lived from 1207 - 1273! In addition to writing poems, Rumi was also recognized as a theologian, legal advisor and spiritual master.

His poems and quotes have been translated into countless languages because he speaks from the heart, which we all understand.

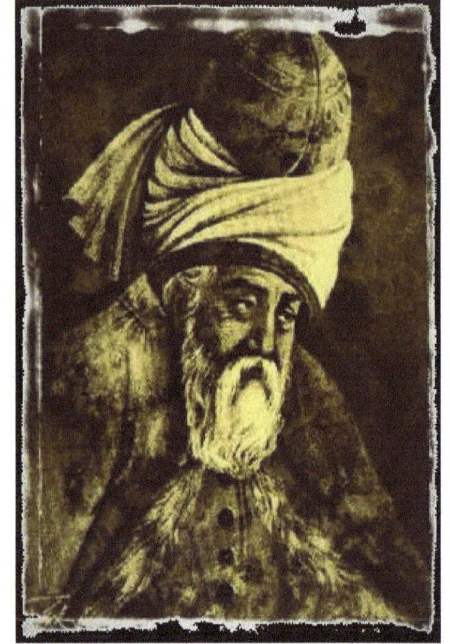

Quotes from Rumi that force me to self-reflection

If you are looking for a friend who is faultless, you will be friendless.

The faults you see in your brother are truly your own, reflected back to you.

Quotes from Rumi that give me strength

If you find all your roads and paths blocked, sHe will show you a secret way that no one knows.

What you seek is seeking you.

As you start to walk on the way, the way appears.

The moment you accept what troubles you've been given the door will open.

Live life as if everything is rigged in your favor.

<u>Quotes from Rumi that speak directly to my</u> 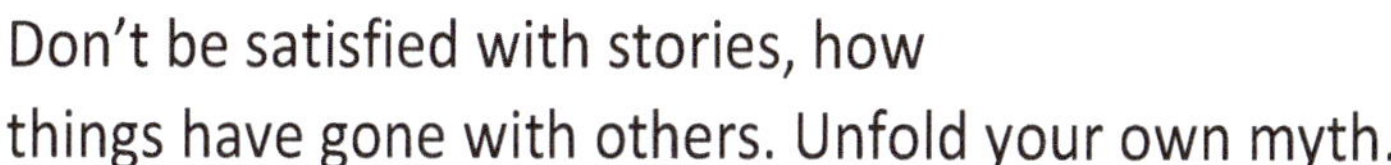

Everyone has been made for some particular work and the desire for that work has been put in every heart.

You have to keep breaking your heart, until it opens.

Be a witness not a judge. Focus on yourself, not on others. Listen to your heart, not to the crowd.

Half of life is lost in charming others. And other half is lost in anxiety caused by others. Leave this game, you have played enough.

Be grateful for whoever comes, because each has been sent as a guide from beyond.

<u>Quotes from Rumi, the coolest</u>

Run from what's comfortable. Forget safety. Live where you fear to live. Destroy your reputation. Be notorious.

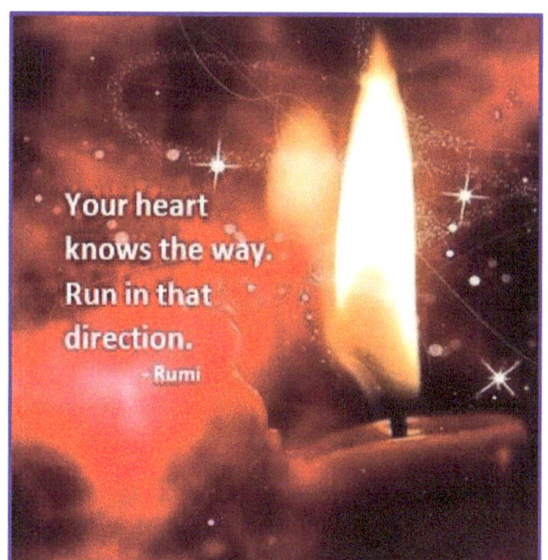

Don't be satisfied with stories, how things have gone with others. Unfold your own myth.

Stop trying to fit in, when you were born to stand out.

I learned that every mortal will taste death. Only some will taste life.

I drink a lot of tea, and love every aspect of tea, partly because of the great taste universe that goes with it 😊

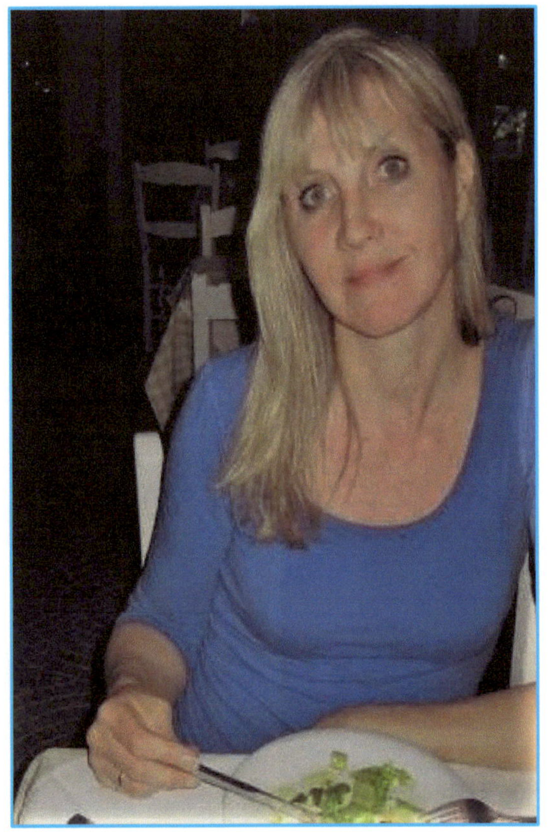

My passion for tea started, in fact, with coffee. I drank a lot of coffee once. When I was in my late 20's, I started getting heartburn, every single time I took a cup of coffee. This is one of the reasons I developed a passion for tea.

Besides my great passion for tea, I care a lot about the environment, animal welfare, human rights and gender equality. I've been a vegetarian for 15 years.

I've lived in Copenhagen for 25 years, and 15 of them, I've shared with Mogens.

When not drinking tea, I enjoy blogging, traveling to exotic places, reading, going to exciting talks, visiting friends and I dream of walking the Camino.

FYI: I also drink wine and champagne.

My very best greetings,

Christie Elene Mogensen